Ten (10) Day Quick Success Weight Loss Program

"A new approach to losing weight by changing your eating habits for life"

I0439994

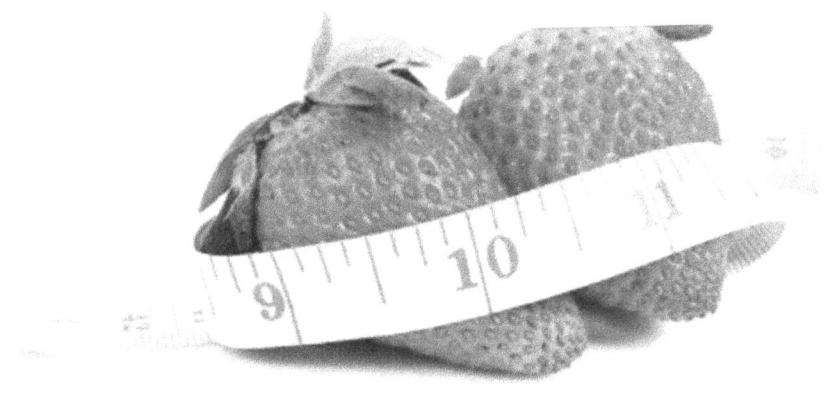

Rudy S. Silva, Natural Nutritionist

Table of Contents

Chapter 1: What Is Weight Loss All About?

What Is Your Reason For Wanting To Lose Weight?

Most of you that are reading this e-book are looking for a quick and safe way to lose weight. Could it be that you are getting married, going to a reunion, getting ready for dating, meeting the new potential mother-in-law?

Most people that are overweight have different reasons for wanting to lose weight. For some it's to look good and to attract the opposite sex. For others it could be to stop the ridicule and gross comments receive daily. And yet for some others, it could be to stop some of the illnesses that favor obesity.

But for whatever reason you have for wanting to trim down, what you will walk away with when you get into this eating habit program, you will weigh less and you will have some of the best health you have ever had.

Losing weight, you have found, is not easy, so you need a diet or an eating habit that you can keep using after your diet period is over.

When you strive to gain the best health you have ever had, you will lose weight. Excess weight and health do not go together. When you have too much weight on your body, you are over working all the organs in your body and reducing their life time. What this does is encourage disease that doesn't necessarily show up right away, but shows up as you age.

Most people over 40 and even sooner start to experience disease that require a doctor's intervention, hospitalization, or drug therapy. If you are overweight, expect this type of life, as time passes.

Is It Your Fault That You Are Overweight?

Being overweight has many causes and sometimes it may not be your fault that you are overweight. If you have a genetic marker that predisposes you to excess weight, then the information here will help you to control your own life.

If you come from an overweight family that allowed you to over eat junk and fatty foods for your meals, then you need to work as an adult to reverse those eating habits that you now have.

If you have thyroid issues, then your metabolism maybe altered, causing you to gain weight. Before you start this program, you might want to get your thyroid function checked.

Now, there are many cases where it is your fault that you are overweight. You decide what food that you want and need to eat. If you are eating more calories than you need, to keep your body working as it should, those calories will be stored as excess fat.

How to Lose Weight

Most people that are overweight eat the wrong kind of food. The food they eat does not provide them with the right nutrition and energy. They over eat fattening food, over cooked food, processed food, fast food, and food in packages and cans.

All of these types of food are high in calories, but lack the right nutrients that the body needs. When you eat food, you should be aware of which foods are high in calories so that you don't eat more calories than your body needs.

High calorie foods should be eaten in small amounts. Low calorie foods should be eaten in larger amounts.

This program does not require you to count calories, but you need to be of aware of those high calorie foods.

Protein – To lose weight, you need to eat good protein. You may not need to eat more than 2 ounces of meat or 60 gm. per day. Your protein needs will depend on the type of work you do. If you are an office worker, are short and have a small body frame, you may only need 1 or 2 oz. of meat per day. But if you are a husky man with a large bone structure and have a physical job, then you may need 12 oz. of meat per day or more.

Quality protein is going to give you the vitality and energy your body needs. The amino acids in the protein will provide the amines needed to create the enzymes you need to control your cell metabolism properly. Good cell metabolism is needed, so that you can control your weight.
Any weight loss program that limits meat from your diet will fail to help you lose weight and to keep it off.

Fiber – By adding the right amount and quality fiber to this eating habit program, you bring in a new factor to losing weight. The combination of protein and quality fiber at each meal will improve your success in losing weight with this eating habit program.

Fiber does not contain calories. It is an indigestible nutrient that exists in carbohydrates that gives you bulk, a feeling of fullness, and helps you lose weight.

Weight loss – You can expect to lose from 5 to 10 lbs. in this 10 day weight loss program. If you continue this eating habit program past 10 day, you will continue to lose more weight. From that point on you will determine how much weight to lose, by the way you eat.

Disease - This eating habit program is good for even people that are not interested in losing weight, but want to slow down the progression of disease, eliminate certain diseases or to gain better overall health.

If you have constipation, this health program will eliminate it. If you have diabetes, this program will help you stabilize your sugar levels. If you have acid reflux or arthritis, this program will help you decrease your symptoms or even eliminate these conditions. This goes to show how critical it is to be the correct weight and eat those foods that give you nutrition and vitality.

This program is designed so that you can flush out toxins that are through out your body and deep into your cell structures. If you have high or low blood pressure, your pressure will start to stabilize. If you suffer from diabetes and many other illnesses, this program will help you reduce the effects of these illnesses.

So how can such an eating habits program produce all of these results? When you move to following a more natural way of eating and living, then the illnesses that you have created will lessen. With this success eating habits program, you can also expect to move to your natural weight.

In this program, you will be eating protein from fish, chicken, and red meat. You need to eat the right amount of meat to lose weight. But you also have to reduce the amount of high calorie carbohydrates. Then, you have to eat the special basic soup, vegetables, fruits, nuts, grains and brown rice listed here.

This special eating habits program combines some of the best information on how to lose weight and how to have a healthy body at the same time. It is based on eating in a way that is natural and in a way that has been used by those civilizations that seldom have obesity and that live to be over 100 years.

Chapter 2: Colon Blood Cleanse

One of the first things you need to do to get started on your weight loss program is to do a two to three day colon and blood cleanse. This is an important step because you want to remove toxins and mucus from your intestinal tract – stomach, small intestine, and colon. In this three day cleanse you will also remove toxins from within your cells and lymph liquid.

This cleanse will also clean out your blood and neutralize many of the acids in your body that are causing you harm. The cleanse will also pull out excess body water and reduce any edema that you might have. This will happen because this cleanse promotes urination and bowel movements.

The combination of toxins, acid, and water can weight from 5 to 7 lbs. or more. This colon and blood cleanse is a great way to start losing weight. You can do this cleanse for two day, but if you do it for three days you will benefit more. It is not that hard to do it for three days.

Constipation

Part of this cleanse is to help you have regular bowel movements. If you do not have one to two bowel movements per day, your body will become toxic. Some toxins are often converted to fat. Keeping regular helps to keep your body clear of toxins and helps to keep your weight down.

To help you clear out your colon there are two ways to do this in this cleanse. You can take Oxypowder during your three day cleanse or you can drink prune juice every day.

In this cleanse, you will only be drinking vegetable juices, fruit juices and eating some fruits for three days. Doing a juice cleanse can give you some side effects, where you feel nausea or slightly sick.

Not everyone will get these effects. If you feel sick, this is a sign that you are stirring up toxins in your stomach and elsewhere in your body, and as you get rid of these toxins you will begin to feel better.

In her extensive book, Cooking For Healthy Healing, 1991, Linda Rector-page, N.D., Ph.D., talks about what a fast does,

"Fasting works by self-digestion. During a cleanse, the body in its infinite wisdom, will decompose and burn only the substances and tissue that are damaged, diseased, or unneeded, such as abscesses, tumors, excess fat deposits, and congestive wastes. Even a relatively short fast can accelerate elimination from the liver, kidneys, lungs and skin, often causing dramatic changes as masses of accumulated waste is expelled. Live foods and juices can literally pick up dead matter from the body and carry it away."

So, here's what you need to do to get started.

The Day Before The Cleanse

Buy the following juices for this cleanse a few days before or the day before your cleanse.

Organic apple juice – one gallon
Organic apples – 3 for one day, 10 apples for three days
Organic prune juice – 1/2 gallon
Organic Cherry juice – 1/2 gallon
Carrots for your juicer or carrot juice – one quart

The day before the fast, eat a large salad and two apples at dinner time. This will give you plenty of fiber to scrub the walls of your colon as you move fecal matter out of your colon the following day.

Cleansing The Colon

If you chose to use Oxy-Powder, then here is where you can buy it on the internet:

Get Oxy-Powder

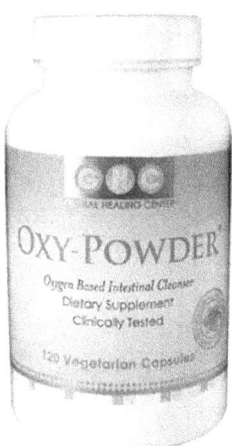

The night before you start your weight loss program, take four Oxy-Powder capsules. If you need to lose a lot of weight, then take five capsules the night before and just before you go to bed.

Now, Oxy-Powder is not a laxative so they are not addictive. What these capsules do is supply oxygen to your colon, which dissolves the hard fecal matter that has built up over time and has not wanted to come out.

Because this bottle of Oxy-Powder has 125 capsules, you can take 1 to 3 capsules during your 10 day weight loss program.

Oxy-Powder causes your stools to become watery, since it is dissolving the hard matter in your colon. Don't be concern that you have diarrhea like symptoms. Also this three day cleanse will also cause you to have watery stools, since you are on a diet of juices and fruits.

If you chose to use prune juice to clear out your colon, this procedure will be described below.

First day of colon cleanse

Do this cleanse on a Saturday, Sunday or any other day that you don't have to go anywhere. You may be going to the bathroom all day and at times you need to be there quick. But, you can do this cleanse even during a work day.

This first morning, you will have a bowel movement when you wake up, because of the Oxy-Powder. After that, go do your lemon drink.

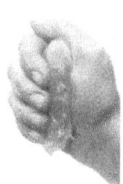 Lemon Juice Drink - Every morning when you first get up, drink a glass of slightly warm water with the juice of 1/2 lemon. This will remove mucus from your intestinal tract and detoxify your liver.

Prune Juice Colon Cleanse

If you decided to use prune juice to clean out your colon, instead of Oxy-Powder, then here is what you need to do.

But you can also do prune juice, if you have done the Oxy-powder since the prune juice is filled with minerals and nutrients that will cleanse your body.

About 1/2 hour after your lemon drink, take 8 oz. of prune juice.

10 minutes later drink another 8 oz. of prune juice
10 minutes later again drink another 8 oz. of prune juice
wait 20 minutes than drink 8 oz. of apple juice
wait 30 minutes than drink another 8 oz. of apple juice

If you haven't sped to the bathroom yet, you will in a little while.

Now drink 8 oz. of apple juice every hour until the end of the day. You can stop drinking apple juice around 5pm. You can use different fruit juices or vegetable juices in place of apple juice, but, just make sure you drink mostly apple juice.

During the day you can eat 1 or 2 apple in the morning and 1 in the evening.

Second Day Of The Colon Cleanse

During the second day, you can drink different kinds of juices and eat 2-6 apples. You can drink any kind of juice be it fruit or vegetable. A combination of fruit and vegetable juice is good. You can add other fruits to eat such as watermelon, melon, oranges, and strawberries.

Third Day Of The Colon Cleanse

The third day is like the second day where you can drink different kinds of juice and eat 2-6 apples or other fruit.

On this day you can eat other fruit like mango, watermelon, cantaloupe, and pineapple. At the end of this day, you can eat a salad with a variety of vegetables.

Fourth Day Start Of Colon Cleanse

You can continue to use Oxy powder at 2 capsules every night for the rest of the month.

Now you ready to start your weight loss program, so let's get stated.

Chapter 3: Helping Your Body Lose Weight

Natural Body Cycles

Your body has natural cycles where it performs various body functions at certain times, such as digestion, detoxifying, and elimination. If you interfere with these cycles, you suppress these functions and this leads to increase weight and disease.

To lose weight and to keep it off, you need to become familiar with your body's natural cycles. You need to eat in a certain way, during these cycles, so that you assist your body in performing its functions.

By learning how to assist your "Body's Natural Cycles", you will be in tune with what your body is doing to eliminate fecal matter from the colon and toxic wastes from your lymph liquid and blood.

Getting in tune with your Natural Body Cycles requires change in the way you eat. Since all of us are addicted to the way we eat, it is, sometimes, difficult to change these habits. But, this is the best information I have found that will give you great health and keep you at your normal weight.

Here are the 3 natural body cycles:

Cycle 1 time period: 4 a.m. to 12 noon

This cycle is the time where your body is eliminating toxins, acids, wastes, and derby through urine, bowel movements, and other secretions. Most people interfere with this cycle, since they are unaware of it, causing constipation, increase weight and various detrimental illnesses.

Cycle 2 time period: 12 noon to 8 p.m.

This is the time when your body should be taking in food and digesting it. By eating the right kind of food, you help your digestive process in your stomach and small intestine. This is your first and second meal of the day – lunch and dinner.

Cycle 3 time period: 8 p.m. to 4 a.m.

This is the time your body is absorbing and using food you have eaten from 12 noon to 8 p.m. Various organs are detoxifying and producing waste and moving it into your kidney and colon. When you wake up, this is the waste you should be getting rid during body cycle one.

The First Body Cycle

During the elimination cycle, 4 a.m. to 12 noon, eat and drink only fruits and their juices or drink vegetable juices. For breakfast, eat a bowl of fruit or have a fruit smoothie made with apple juice, banana, and fruits in season.

Before noontime, eat fruits as snacks. Forty-five minutes before noon eat your last fruit. You can eat and drink all the fruits and juices you want up to noontime.

Fruits contain the right balance of nutrients with about 70% distilled water. Eat them without cooking them. They are easy to digest and absorb and do not stress your colon. They activate peristaltic action in your colon and help you have a bowel movement.

Here are some of the fruits to eat:

Apples
Apricots
Avocados

Bananas
Blueberries
Boysenberries
Cantaloupes
Cherries
Figs and dates
Grapes
Grapes
Lemons
Nectarines
Oranges
Papayas
Peaches
Pears
Persimmons
Plums
Prunes
Raspberries
Strawberries
Watermelons

Eat all melons together and not with other fruit and wait 1/2 hour before eating other fruit. Melons require specific enzymes to be digested in the stomach, so other fruit eaten with melons will just sit in your stomach, waiting to be digested and can cause gas and an acid stomach.

By eating fruits during body cycle 1 you are assisting your body's elimination cycle. Fruits and juices help your body to urinate, or have a bowel movement, and eliminate toxins and acids from your body and blood. It is these toxins and acids that make you, overweight, constipated, and sick.

Eating solid food for breakfast – eggs potatoes, rice, meat, cereal, milk, and so on, the typical breakfast, interferes with your body's elimination cycle and eventually leads to sickness and excess weight.

It takes over 3 hours to digest heavy and solid food. The food you should be eating in the morning should digest quickly. This helps you to activate peristaltic colon action to create a bowel movement and to continue your body's detoxification and elimination process.

Heavy food slows down the elimination of toxins from your body and this causes chime and toxins to remain in your colon longer than necessary. These toxins then get stored in your body as fat and acids.

Acids are the main cause of most illnesses, so you want to have an alkaline body. Fruits and vegetables neutralize acids and give you an alkaline body. An alkaline body is the healthiest body condition you can have.

It takes 1 to 1 1/2 hour or so to digest fruits and fruit juices. Because of this, they help to cleanse your body of waste during the time from 4am to noontime.

So if you are not already having fruit and fruit and vegetables juices for breakfast and snacks, start slowing changing your eating habits, if you want to lose weight and feel better.

The Second Natural Body Cycle

Here is the second body cycle and it occurs from 12 noon to 8 p.m.

This is the time when your body should be taking in food and digesting it. During this period it is time to eat solid food. What you eat has to be in alignment with what your stomach can do.

Here's how your stomach works. In generally it can only digest one solid food at a time.

A solid food is one that does not contain 70% water, like fruits and vegetables do, and whose water has been eliminated by heat or other food processes, in other words cooked.

Your stomach can only work on one solid food at a time, so your lunch and dinner should only have one solid food. A lunch can consist of chicken and a green salad, fish and a green salad, tuna and a green salad, shrimp and a green salad, beef and a green salad.

Mixing a protein meal with carbohydrates is giving the stomach two solid foods at the same time, which require different concentrations of digestive juices.

When you eat any animal protein, avoid eating it with nonstarchy vegetables - artichokes, yams, sweet potatoes, carrots, oats, peas, potatoes, rice, wheat, winter squash and corn. These vegetables breakdown into sugars that coat your protein food and this causes a chemical process called glycation, which creates inflammation and lowers your immunity. In addition, this combination of protein and starches are difficult to digest and disrupt your second body cycle.

When you eat animal protein eat it with broccoli, cabbage, cauliflower, celery, cucumber, garlic, green beans, leafy greens onions, garlic, wakame, dulse, and zucchini.

Giving the stomach more than it can handle interrupts the elimination cycle 1 and reduces the energy that you need for the elimination cycle.

Any eating habits that disrupts cycle 2, the eating and digestion cycle, affects the other cycles. Here's how you can help your body's cycle 2 to be more effective.

1. Eat only one solid food with vegetables during lunch or dinner. Lunch can be one meat or seafood with a fresh vegetable salad that is nonstarchy.

2. Or you can eat only brown or red rice or other grains, with both starchy and nonstarchy vegetables, with no

3. Limit the amount of water you drink during meals. Excess water will dilute your digestive acids and slow down digestion of your food.

4. Avoid drinking sodas, tea or other drinks during your meals. If you need to clear your dry throat, use room temperature water. Cold liquids will slow down your digestive processes.

5. Eating meals with more than one solid food such as meat and potatoes, chicken and rice, fish and rice, chicken and noodles, eggs and toast, cheese and bread will diminish the energy you need during the elimination cycle

6. It is permissible to eat beef and chicken at the same time but not chicken and eggs or beef and nuts or chicken and beans. Eat the same type of protein at the same time, but do not mix different proteins.

7. It's ok to eat different types of carbohydrates at the same time, with a salad, but not with protein, since carbohydrates digest easier than protein.

Eating a variety of food at the same time leads to undigested food. Food that is partially undigested becomes acidic, which affects the health of your colon and causes constipation. When these acids are absorbed into your body, they are converted into fat and stored as toxins your body.

Eating the right combination of foods at meal time, helps you to preserve your energy for the elimination cycle and prevents you from creating spoiled food in your stomach that is converted to acid waste. It is this acid waste that results in illness and fat. This is the reason most people as they age come down with various illnesses that terminate their life early or gain excessive weight.

The Third Body Cycle

The third body cycle is the assimilation cycle and is from 8pm to 4am. This is the time the food you have eaten during the day is assimilated, absorbed and distributed throughout your body through your blood. It is the time where digested food moves into the colon as chime and is stored there for elimination. And, you should be eliminating this chime or fecal matter, when you wake up or during the morning to 12 noon.

Food eaten during the second cycle, 12 noon to 8 p.m. and that was combined and eaten properly will digest within 3 to 4 hours, whereas food not combine properly, a meal consisting of protein and carbohydrates will take up to 8 hours to pass through your stomach. During this time, your food will putrefy and ferment and become acidic. Under these conditions, you will not get many nutrients from that meal.

So, eat your last meal by 6-7 pm, so that your food digests in your stomach by the time you go to bed. After three hours later, your food will have moved into your small intestine where it is ready for assimilation.

When you go to bed 3 hours after your last meal, the next 6 hours, until 4am, your body will be absorbing the food you have eaten the previous day and moving waste into your colon.

Remember, anything you do different than what these cycles call for will disrupt them and cause them to become extended and your cycle time will be off.

Just start changing your eating habits slowly and as time passes you will be doing more and more of what your body's natural cycles need.

Chapter 4: Success Weight Loss Principles

Here is an outline of what you need to do to lose the weight you want. This is the 10 day weight loss eating habits program and you can lose from to 7 to 14 lbs. during this time. And if you continue this program after 10 days you can continue to lose weight, even with a relaxed success eating habits program.

Principles of this eating habits program

The basic principles of this program are to eat foods from the six food groups as identified below:

Carbohydrate Food

Starchy foods
Fruits and their juices
Milk and yogurt

Non Carbohydrate Food

Non starchy vegetables
Protein
Fats

Quantity of food that you eat is important to control and to make sure that the food you eat has plenty of fiber. In this program there is no need to count calories, but the amount of calories you eat is important. You need to avoid eating high calories foods in excess. You can eat them but in small quantities.

It is just common sense that if you consume more calories

than you need to run your body during the day, then the excess calories you eat will be converted into fat.

You will be given a set of charts that tells you which foods you need to eat the most of to lose weight. What you will be concentrating on is eating the amount of food from the given list in an amount that does not exceed your energy requirements.

Even better, is to eat the amount of food that does not provide the calories you need for your daily requirements. When you do this, your body will look to use the fat you have stored, to provide the extra calories you need.

You can eat less food and exercise to use up some of your body fat. Your body will provide that calories from your body fat, when you don't eat enough food to provide your body with the calories it needs for that day. If you exercise in addition to eating less, you will burn up more body fat.

All this is fine in theory and many diets use these principles, yet people lose weight and gain it back after they finish their diet?

The basis Of This Eating Habits Program

What is outlined in this program is a way to eat using the **body cycles** and eating foods from all food groups in certain quantities that will become your way of eating all of the time. This provides you with a way of losing weight and then relaxing on some the rules provided after your weight program, so that you can eat other foods you like and still lose small amounts of weight or maintain your weight.

One of the main principles is to eat from all food groups – **protein, carbohydrates, dairy, and fats** - small amounts, so that you don't feel deprived of these foods and cause you to beige on these foods, when you finish your program.

The other principle is to eat those foods with **high fiber** content, so that you can up your fiber content from around 12 gm. to 30 to 35 gm.

Eating more fiber foods, which are lower in calories, is important in this program. When you eat fiber foods, you feel filled, so you eat less. You need to eat fiber foods at all meals. The food charts provided will show you which foods are the highest in fiber. These foods are typically fruits and vegetables.

Fiber also provides bulk that slows down your digestion in the small intestine and thereby reducing the amount of sugar, fat, and toxins that enter your body. The result is some of this excess digested food is routed to the colon where it is also held in the feces, which is later disposed of in your stools.

Fiber is also one of the nutrients that keeps you healthy. It is a key in reducing your susceptibility to cardiovascular, diabetes, and colon diseases.

Glycogen

All carbohydrates are converted to glucose during digestion. Here's how the conversion occurs

Starchy foods contain maltose
Fruits and their juices contain fructose
Milk and yogurt contain lactose

Maltose, fructose and lactose are converted to glucose. In the liver glucose is converted to glycogen. This glycogen is stored in the liver and in muscle tissue. When your body is low in glucose, glycogen is released from the liver and converted to glucose to cover the shortage. Your body runs on glucose and your cells convert it to energy.

Only a certain amount of glycogen can be stored in the liver and muscle tissues. When these areas are filled, the excess coming in from the food you eat is converted to fat and stored though out your body.

So it is not carbohydrates that cause fat, but it's eating an excess of carbohydrates or an excess of any other food that causes fat. The solution is to eat less food of all kinds and exercise regularly.

Your liver can only store 100 gm. of glycogen every day. Your muscles can store 250 to 400 grams of glycogen. Your overall average of glycogen that you can store daily is around 260 gm.

The muscles will not use up glycogen when your organs or cells need it, except in an emergency. Glycogen in the muscles is used to provide you energy for exercising or for fight or flight situations.

Chapter 5: Success Weight Loss Program – Basic Soup

Ok, now that you have some tools and concepts to use in your weight loss program, now we can get into the details of this program. You will be eating vegetables, fruits, juices, protein, fiber, fats, brown rice or red rice, fish, chicken, red meat, and soup. You can eat white rice if you don't have brown or red rice, but limit the amount you eat.

You will use smoothies, fruit puddings, fruits juices, and vegetable juices, whole fruits and raw vegetables. When you make the soup describe here you can eat this soup all day long and in this way you will not feel hungry.

In this program, you will be eating the following:

Protein – The best protein to eat is found in fish. So eat fish as often as you can. Eat the fish for lunch and not for dinner. Serve yourself up to 2 to 4 oz. per meal and don't over eat protein, because what your body does not use, it will be stored as fat.

Vegetables – Always eat vegetables with your meat. This provides the fiber you need to help the digested meat flow easier through your colon. The more vegetables you eat the less hungry you will be after each meal. Eat your vegetables raw when possible and if cooked, use a small amount of water at the bottom of the pot. Then, cook them for 3 to 4 minutes with a lid over the pot. If your vegetables are over cooked they will be wilted and soft.

Do not use salt in this program, since salt attracts water and this will prevent you from losing the weight that you want.

Also, do not use chilies.

Start of the Eating habits program

First do the 3 day fruit and vegetable colon and blood cleansing diet. This will remove a lot of toxins from your body fluids, blood, and colon. It will remove the excess water and get your body ready for a different type way of eating.

Morning Drink

Each day of the 10 day eating program, start your day with one of the following drinks. Choose one and the next day drink a different one if you like.

1. In 8 oz. of distilled water, squeeze the juice of one lemon. This drink is good for flushing the liver, providing minerals, and eliminating internal mucus.

2. Prepare a cup of green tea and add the juice of one lemon. Green tea is super and is high in antioxidants. It is one of the best drinks for your cardiovascular system.

3. In 8 oz. of distilled water put 1 to 2 tablespoons, even more when you get use to the taste, of liquid chlorophyll, with the juice of one lemon.

4. In 8 oz. of distilled water, add one scoop of your favorite green powder. You can use the Green SuperFood at Amazon.

5. If you are a lite breakfast person, than a glass of juice might be all you need, but you need to eat more so that you don't get hungry before noon. Use any of the fruit juices or vegetable juices listed here. A glass of half orange and grapefruit is a good starter drink. A glass of tomato juice with the juice of one lemon is another. You may already have a favorite juice to drink.

Then consider taking various different juice drinks in a thermos to work for breaks.

Basic Special Soup

Here is a soup that you need to make and use frequently. This is the basic special soup and as you read on you will discover how to make this soup with other vegetables.

To start with you need to get rid of your table salt and not use it. Yes you need sodium but you need to get it from vegetables, which provide organic salt. You can use other spices to make your soup and food tasteful.

Make this soup with these vegetables, which will help you reduce weight. These vegetable take more energy to eat than the energy they give you, yet they will provide you with the nutrients you need to move your body to alkaline and to keep you healthy.

Cut the following vegetables into small to medium sizes and place them into a big pot. You want to make enough soup to last for a couple of days. The unused portion you can refrigerate.

5-6 onions
2-3 cloves of garlic
Medium size cabbage head
One bunch of celery
One small green and one small red pepper
One can of whole or cut tomatoes
A cupful or less of mixed chili power to your taste

Cover the vegetables with water and boil water for ten minutes, then simmer for 2-3 hours.

This soup is designed to keep you feeling full and is not to provide a lot of nutrition. You can eat this soup all day long since it will not make you gain weight. What you can do is put it in a thermos and take it to work and eat it wherever you are.

This soup is used to eat between meals as a snack. You will also be using fruit juices and fruits to eat as snacks.

Other Soup Vegetables

Here are more vegetables that you can add to your base soup so that you have variation of this soup for different days. In addition, use these vegetable to make some of your salads. Many of these vegetables also require more energy to digest and absorb than they give you.

NONSTRACHY VEGETABLES LIST

Each vegetable listed below is a serving of ½ cup cooked or 1 cup raw. The numbers to the right are the fiber content of each vegetable in grams.

Vegetables	Fiber (gm.)
Artichoke	6
Artichoke Hearts	4
Asparagus	3
Bean Sprouts	1
Beets	2
Broccoli	2
Brussels Sprouts	2
Cabbage	2
Carrots	2
Cauliflower	2
Celery	1
Cucumber	1
Eggplant	2
Green Onions Or Scallions	1
Greens (Collard, Kale, Mustard, Turnip)	2
Kohlrabi	2
Leeks	1
Mixed Vegetables (Without Corn, Peas)	1

Mushrooms	1
Okra	2
Onions	1
Pea Pods	2
Peppers	1
Salad Greens	1
Spinach	2
Summer Squash	4
Tomato	1
Tomato Sauce	2
Tomato/Vegetable Juice	1
Turnips	2
Water Chestnuts	1
Water Cress	1
Zucchini	1

If you want zucchini with 2 grams of fiber, you would have to eat 1 cup of cooked zucchini.

Choose from this list of vegetable when preparing your soups and all three meals. Try to choose those vegetables that will give you a total of 30 to 35 grams of fiber each day.

Remember that you need to eat up to 30 to 35 grams per day so that you can start to lose weight. You can eat all the vegetables you want that are on this list. You cannot get fat eating these vegetables.

Chapter 6: Success Weight Loss Program- Eating Breakfast

During the period from the time you wake up to noon time, you can drink tea and eat only fruits and vegetables. When you first wake up here's what to do.

Drink one glass of water with half the juice of one lemon.

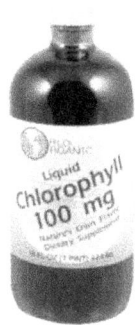

30 minutes later drink a green drink in one of two ways. You can put 1 to 2 tablespoons of liquid chlorophyll in 8 oz. of water or a capful of your favorite green powder in 8 oz. of water.

For the **chlorophyll drink**, add the juice of 1/2 lemon juice to give it some flavor. For the **green power** drink, add some honey so it is easier to drink.

After Your Morning Drink

After you finish your morning drink wait about 1/2 hour before you start your breakfast. Eat only fruits for breakfast. Choose from any of these fruit preparations and choose different ones during the 10 days.

Eating fruits and drinking only juices from morning to noon is part of the body cycle I process. It's in the morning that you help your body to eliminate body toxins that have accumulated during the night. Since fruits and juices have a short digestion cycle, this cycle helps you to better eliminate waste from your body every morning.

Here are a few morning breakfast suggestions:

1. Cut and prepare a bowl of various fresh fruits. Do not add any toppings.

2. Cut and mix watermelon and cantaloupe slices together. Do not mix this fruit with other types of fruit.

3. Prepare a fruit pudding in a blender using 3 or 4 different fruits listed in the previous chapter. This is a great way to get plenty of nutrients into your body fast. It also fills and satisfies your hunger. Use different fruits or use the same ones for a few days. You can add a touch of honey, lecithin, or different juices to adjust the consistency of the pudding.

    You can prepare a mango, pineapple, strawberry, banana, apple, peach, and apricot pudding. Just experiment with the different fruit puddings you can prepare.

    You can put some of this pudding in a thermos and use it for snacks during the morning or afternoon break.

4. Prepare your base soup as described in the previous chapter. You can prepare this the previous day and all you have to do is heat it up in the morning. Also take a thermos of this soup to work and you can eat this all day long, if you like. This soup is non-fatting and will keep your hunger at bay.

5. Prepare a smoothie as shown in the smoothie chapter. Drink part of it for breakfast and the rest for your breaks.

6. On occasion you can eat a pouched egg or a small amount of whole oats, not the quick cooking oats. You can use apple juice to dilute the oats and add a banana and raisins. You can do this once a week, if you like.

Fruit Pudding

Next mix a fruit pudding to take to work for a snack. Here are two different things you can do with a blender. Take these blended fruits to work in a thermos to eat when you get there.

Put into a blender

Two small or one large banana
One mango
Pineapple
One apple
1/4 of a papaya (if available)
Small amount of apple juice to make this blend into a pudding

Blend all of this for 1 – 2 minutes.

You can add lecithin granules or powdered vitamin C to make it more a tart and to preserve it.

Pineapple Smoothie

Mix the following in a blender to create a smoothie. In a later chapter you will find some addition smoothie recipes.

1-2 cups of fresh pineapples
1/2 cups apple slices
1/4 cup fresh apple juice
1/4 cup rice dream (more or less as needed)
1 small banana
1-teaspoon lecithin
1-teaspoon flax seed oil
2 teaspoons bran (oat or rice)
1/2 of plain yogurt

You can alternate using the pudding and smoothie during the 10 days. Also you can change the fruit from pineapples to mango or strawberries. More smoothie recipes are in another chapter. Don't use a smoothie every day. Use the smoothie to break the monotony of eating only sliced fruits.

Now about 1/2 hour or so before lunch eat some of the basic soup. Do this every day of your 10 day weight loss time. You can also use the basic soup as an afternoon snack.

Morning Snack time

During your morning and afternoon break, it's time to open your thermos and have a good snack. Make sure you take your snack break. Use only fruits, vegetables, nuts, and soups for your snacks. These types of snacks help you to digest your food better and also activate peristaltic colon action. They give you fiber and many of the minerals you need to make your body more alkaline.

To make your body more alkaline, use fresh fruits such as grapes, apples, watermelon, cantaloupes, apricots, peaches, pineapples, strawberries, other berries, mangos, and so on. Check the Alkaline Chapter 8 for the fruits to eat.

Use drinks like apple, cherry, prune, pineapple, tomato, carrot, and so on. Review the chapter on fruits.

There you have it, the breakfast. Do this every morning for the 10 days. After 10 day, continue eating in the manner, but in a more relax way. This should become your new eating habit.

Fruit and Fiber

Here is a list of fruits that give you the most fiber. Try to get up to 30 to 35 grams of fiber every day. If you are short on fiber for the day look at this list of fruits and eat the ones that give you more fiber. Also notice the fruit serving and if you want more fiber double the serving.

FRUIT LIST	Fruit Serving	Fiber
Apple, unpeeled, small	1 (4 oz.)	4
Applesauce, unsweetened	½ cup	1
Apples, dried	4 rings	2

Food	Serving	Value
Apricots, fresh	4 whole	1
Apricots, dried	8 halves	4
Apricots, canned	½ cup	1
Banana, small	1 (4 oz.)	1
Blackberries	¾ cup	5
Blueberries	¾ cup	5
Cantaloupe, small	1 cup cubes	2
Cherries, fresh	12	2
Cherries, sweet, canned	½ cup	1
Dates	3	2-3
Figs, dried	2	2
Fruit cocktail	½ cup	1
Grapefruit, large	½	1
Grapes	17	1
Honeydew melon	1 slice	1
Kiwi	1	3
Mandarin oranges, canned	¾ cup	1
Mango, small	½ cup	1
Nectarine, small	1	2
Orange, small	1 (6 ½ oz.)	3
Papaya	½ fruit	3 Peach, fresh
	1	2
Peaches, canned	½ cup	1
Pear, large, fresh	½ (4 oz.)	4
Pears, canned	½ cup	1
Pineapple, fresh	¾ cup	1
Pineapple, canned	½ cup	1
Plums, small	2	2
Raisins	2 tbsp.	1
Raspberries	1 cup	8
Strawberries	1 ¼ cup	4
Tangerines, small	2	2
Watermelon	1 ¼ cup	1

Juice To Drink

Here are the juices to drink during your break time or for your smoothies. You can drink many of the other juices listed in the other chapters, especially for your smoothies. You can also make fresh juices with these fruits in a juicer. When you do, include some of the pulp in your juice to get some fiber.

FRUIT JUICE, UNSWEETENED Fiber	SERVING
Apple juice/cider	½ cup
Cranberry juice cocktail	1/3 cup
Cranberry juice cocktail, reduced-calorie	1 cup
Fruit juice blends, 100% juice	1/3 cup
Grape juice	1/3 cup
Grapefruit juice	½ cup
Orange juice	½ cup
Prune juice	1/3 cup

Chapter 7: Success Weight Loss Program – Lunch And Dinner

You will be using brown rice for your lunch or dinner. Brown rice has protein, B vitamin, and many minerals that you need. According to the George Mateljan Foundation, one cup of brown rice has:

"216 calories, or 12 percent of the daily value (DV). It also is an excellent source of manganese, a trace mineral, providing 88 percent DV, and a good source of selenium and magnesium, providing 27.3 percent and 21 percent DV, respectively. A cup of this rice also contains protein (10.06 percent DV), carbohydrates (14.92 percent DV) and dietary fiber (14.04 percent DV)."

You can also use red rice. Like brown rice, it has more fiber and nutritional value than white rice. It also takes longer to cook than white rice. If you don't like brown rice try the red rice or use the white rice but not as much as you usually eat.

How To Cook Brown Rice or Red Rice

Use the following ingredients.

1 cup natural brown rice or red rice
8 cups cold water (you can also only 4 to 5 cups of water. What you want is to have a lot of water over your rice after you have cooked the rice for the time mention below.)

Rinse rice for 30 seconds or so to clean it out. Boil water first in a large pot with a lid and then add the rice. Lower the heat, so that that water still has a strong boil, but does not cause an overflow of water.

Keep the lid slightly open so that steam does not overflow. Stir in the rice and cook on medium heat for 30 minutes. You can experiment with this time. You can try 25 minutes or 35 minutes. In different parts of the country the time will be slightly different.

Drain or pour the water out of the pot. Move the pot and rice with cover to a different place to let it cool for 20 minutes more. No heat is necessary since the heat of the pot and rice will finish the cooking. This will make between 3 to 4 cups of cooked rice.

You can take this rice to work and place the extra in a closed container into the refrigerator for the following days.

You can eat as much of the brown rice that you want and you might want to add it to your soup on some days. But do not mix meat into your soup when you add rice to it.

Lunch time

For lunch you want to make sure you have a salad that has the vegetables listed in the previous chapters. And, make sure you include the dark green leafy lettuce, tomato, cucumber, and celery.

Meat

You can chose any meat that you want, such as ground lean meat, filet mignon, T-bone, sirloin, tenderloin, lamb, veal. Don't over load on the meat you only need a couple of ounces.

If you like fish, this is the best protein you can eat. Fish protein takes longer to digest, so it is better to eat it for lunch instead of dinner. Try to eat fish 2 to 3 times a week.

Here is a list of meats you can eat. Use 2 to 3 oz. of meat.

Meat And Meat Substitute List   Serving Size

Poultry: chicken or turkey (white or dark meat,
      No skin), Cornish hen, no skin   1 oz.

Fish: fresh or frozen cod, flounder, haddock,
      Halibut, trout, lox, tuna fish   1 oz.
      (fresh or canned in water)

Shellfish: clams, crab, lobster, scallops, shrimp 1 oz.

Game: duck or pheasant (no skin), venison,
      Buffalo, ostrich   1 oz.

Beef: USDA select or choice grades of lean
    beef trimmed of fat, such as round, sirloin,

    flank steak, tenderloin, roast (rib, chuck,   1 oz.
    rump), steak (T-bone, porterhouse, cubed),
    ground round

Pork: lean pork, fresh ham;
    canned, cured, or boiled ham,
    Canadian bacon, tenderloin,   1 oz.
    center loin chop

Lamb: roast chop or leg   1 oz.

Veal: Lean chop, roast   1 oz.

Fish: herring (uncreamed or smoked)   1 oz.

Oysters   1 oz.

Salmons (fresh or canned), catfish   1 oz.

Sardines (canned)   2 medium
Tuna (canned in oil, drained)

Some Breads that you can eat with meals.

STARCH BREAD LIST

	Serve Size	Fiber
Biscuit, 2 ½ inches across	1	1
Bread, white	1 slice	1
Bread, pumpernickel, rye	1 slice	2
Bread, whole-wheat	1 slice	2-6
Corn bread, 2-inch cube	1 (2 oz.)	1
English muffin	½	1
English muffin, whole-wheat	½	2
Tortilla, corn or flour, 6 inches across	1	1
Tortilla, flour, 10 inches across	¼	1

Rice and Meat

For lunch you can eat brown rice and 4 oz. of meat. This meat can be beef, lamb, veal, chicken, turkey, or fish. Do not fry any of this meat. It is best to bake or broil this meat. Try to eat more fish or sea food than any of the other types of meat. Use a small amount of rice. But it is best to only eat meat with salad, since this will give you the best digestion.

You can also eat cottage cheese with fresh fruit such as pineapples, and a salad with a variety of lettuces and vegetable listed above.

Dinner Time

For dinner you can have rice and fish. It is best to have the same type of protein you had for lunch. This will help you digest your food better. So if you have chicken for lunch have chicken for dinner.

You don't even have to have any meat, or have very little, for dinner and have rice, soup, and salad. Or you can have a cup full of rice and a pouched egg. You can also add some chili sauce into a pan and break an egg into the sauce after it is hot and cook the egg and add it to your brown rice.

If you don't want to have a salad, then cook some vegetables, from the vegetable list, with a little water and just long enough to get them slightly soft.

Fatty Foods

Here is a list of fat you can eat. For a healthy diet you need to eat some fat both saturated and unsaturated. But you have to go easy on eating fat and not go overboard.

In this case, use only the listed amounts with your meals.

Saturated Fat

	Serving Size
Butter, stick	1 tsp.
Butter, reduced-fat	1 tbsp.
Coconut, sweetened, shredded	2 tbsp.
Coconut milk	1 tbsp.
Cream cheese:	
Regular	1 tbsp.
Reduced-fat	1 ½ tbsp.
Sour cream:	
Regular	2 tbsp.
Reduced-fat	3 tbsp.
Avocado, medium	2 tbsp.
Oil (canola, olive, peanut)	1 tsp.
Nuts: almonds cashews,	
mixed (50%peanuts, hazelnuts	6 nuts
Peanuts	10 nuts
Pecans	4 halves
Peanut butter, smooth or crunchy	½ tbsp.
Sesame seeds	1 tbsp.
Seeds: pumpkin, sunflower	1 tbsp.
Nuts: walnuts, pecans, Brazil nuts	4 halves

Drinking Water, Juices, And Eating Fruits

Try not to have any water with your lunch or dinner during

your meal. Drink water or juice about 1/2 or 1 hour after your meal. Drinking any type of liquid with your meal will change your stomach pH and can affect your natural digestion process.

Also do not eat fruits immediately after your meals. Eat them after about 1 hour after meals. Fruits and juices should be used as between meal snacks or for the breakfast.

Drink as least 4 cups of distilled water or ROI water every day. Since you are eating fruits and juices, you are getting plenty more water.

Afternoon Snack Time

You can have any leftover protein as a snack. This is also the time that you should be taking the special vegetable soup that you made earlier. You can also eat fruit or juices that will help make you alkaline. By eating these types of snacks, you will be less hungry during lunch or dinner.

When Hungry

At any time that you feel hungry, you can eat all the special soup and salad you want or you can eat brown rice with vegetables. You can also eat fruits and juices that give you alkaline minerals. But, don't eat fruits and juices with your meals unless they are vegetables juices. Don't drink large quantities of juices, since they are high in fructose, which is converted to excess fat during your digestion.

Near Bed Time

Don't eat 2 to 3 hours before bed time. If you get hungry during this time, drink some juice or have a small portion of fruit such as pineapple or any other fruit.

Desserts You Can Eat

These are the low carbohydrate desserts you can eat.

Fruits

Jell-O or Agar Agar (add banana, berries, cantaloupe, peaches, or pineapple to the Jell-O) no sugar but you can add a touch of honey

Banana Custer without sugar

Banana with skimmed milk

Berries with milk

Apples raw, baked or stewed with some cinnamon on the baked apple

Here is a salad dressing you can make and use on your salads.

Apple cider vinegar
Flax seed oil
Olive oil
Lecithin granules

Use two times more flax seed oil as olive oil. Use apple cider vinegar to your tastes. Use a teaspoon of lecithin to help you digest and absorb these oils better.

Foods To Avoid

These are the foods that will cause you to gain weight and you need to avoid these while on this diet. Later when you are on a maintenance diet you can eat some of these foods but not as much as you did before this diet.

Potatoes
Ice cream
Canned fruits with sugar
Gravies

Mayonnaise
Salad dressings
Baked products such as cakes, pies, cookies, donuts
Alcoholic drinks
Sodas and all sugary drinks
All foods in packages or junk food
All sugary products or desserts
Jelly or jam
Peanut butter
Nuts

You can maintain your weight by eating all of these types of food, but you have to limit the amount of these foods that you eat.

The Secret is that you need to keep your fiber intake to 30 to 35 grams per day, eat plenty of vegetables and protein. You can also eat carbohydrates but you need to limit the amount you eat. Do not eat these foods during your program, but only during your maintenance period.

The food values given in the chart are so you can keep track of how much fiber you eat.

Supplements

If you are taking vitamins, minerals, herbals, or other nutrients, just continue taking them. Take them before or after your meals.

How To Cook Protein

Most beef you should broil. Lamb you should broil or roast. Pork should be broiled or roasted. Poultry should be roasted. Fish should be broil or baked. Shrimp, crab, scallops, clams, or oysters can be fried.

Chapter 8: Foods To Eat For An Alkaline Body

Losing weight and maintaining a healthy body go hand in hand. You cannot be healthy and be overweight. At some point in your life, you will develop a condition or illness that is related to your excess weight or to an acid body.

Of course, not being overweight doesn't mean you are healthy. To be in good health, you need to have a good lifestyle and this means eating and living healthy.

When you eat natural food that gives you good health, your body will be alkaline and this condition produces better health. In this chapter, you will discover what it means to have an acid body and an alkaline body. Then you will see what foods you need to eat to have an alkaline body.

Minerals

Moving your body more toward alkalinity is what will help you lose weight. If you have an acid body, it will be hard to lose weight. An acid body attracts disease, pathogens, and water, which produces toxins that can be stored as fat. In addition, a diseased body is associated with being overweight and lacking the proper nutrition.

An alkaline body prevents your body from becoming ill and forming deadly diseases, like all kinds of joint problems, organ degradation, body pain, heart disease, or even cancer. If you are already sick, then all of the chemicals inside fruits will help to revive you to better health. This is provided that your tissue damage has not gone beyond repair.

The minerals most important in changing and maintaining your body in an alkaline condition are sodium, potassium, chloride, calcium, phosphorus, magnesium, and sulphur.

Now, how your body can become alkaline might become a little confusing at first because of the terms used, but let's break this down into small parts. First we are going to be defining some terms, so we can then start talking the same language

Acid Binding

There are certain minerals that are called acid binding. And these are minerals we said are the most important ones in fruits - Sodium, potassium, chloride, calcium, phosphorus, and magnesium - because they are acid binding.

What acid binding means is when you eat fruits with these minerals, they will combine with acids in your body and neutralize them. These neutralized acids will be then be eliminated from your body in your urine and feces.

If not all the acid toxins are captured by acid binding matter, the remaining acids can be neutralized by body stores of alkaline minerals. If you don't have a good store of alkaline minerals, then these acids will remain in your body creating disease. But if you do have a good store of alkaline minerals, these minerals will find acids, capture them, and bind with them. Then these acids will be moved out of your body, by your urine, stools, and breath.

So you can see the importance of getting a lot of alkaline minerals into your body. Without them, acids would not get eliminate from your body, and they would remain in your body tissue and continue their body damage.

Acid binding minerals mainly come from eating vegetables and fruits.

Alkaline Binding

Now, there are also minerals that become alkaline binding and these minerals are sulphur, chlorine, iodine, phosphorus, bromine, fluorine, copper, and silicon. It is these minerals that when digested by a cell will produce a salt that will bind with alkaline minerals. These minerals will be excreted through your urine.

When alkaline minerals are trapped by an acid salt, the alkaline mineral is removed from your body and your body becomes more acidic. This is the condition you are trying to avoid.

Foods that are alkaline binding and remove the minerals that you need to make your body alkaline are meat, carbohydrates, some vegetables and some fruits.

Although you need to eat both foods that are acid binding or alkaline binding, you want to eat more of the acid binding foods. This will keep your body slightly alkaline.

Where do Acid Toxins Come From?

So why is the body overloaded with toxins? Why can't the liver take care of these toxins? Your liver has the function to remove acid wastes from natural food that is created by food digestion and cell metabolism. When your body encounters acid wastes, such as food enhancers, dyes, preservatives, pesticides, and the variety of additives, the liver does not know how to break them down or make them harmless.

But your body does not give up so easily, when it knows that the liver is not able to disintegrate food additives. What it does is it instructs calcium to bind with these toxic acids and to take them far away from the blood stream.

Now, we have talked about acid toxins in the body that are brought in through food and the environment. But there is another factor that creates acid in the body and that is emotions that are activated through life stresses, like work pressures, divorce, friendship problems, martial issues, and other similar situations. These emotional problems create acidic molecules that then embed themselves into your tissues just like food acids. These again can be removed with minerals.

Body Organs

All body organs function to rid the body of acid waste or toxins. Lack of acid binding food causes the deterioration of these organs. Each organ has a specific function in the elimination and neutralization of acid wastes and it does this in conjunction with acid binding minerals.

Acid Binding Foods

Here is a list of the fruits that have the highest alkaline minerals and the ones that you should be eating to eliminate your body acids.

The percentage assigned to these fruits is based on fresh fruits that are organic and that they are not cooked, canned or mixed with sugar. If they are cook or otherwise processed in some fashion, this will reduce their effectiveness as an acid binding fruit. However, they will still be somewhat effective in acid binding.

Fruits above 50% in value are more acid binding, which means they will trap acid wastes better. You will want to eat and drink those fruits above 51%.

The fruits that are at 50% at are neutral. They are not acid binding nor alkaline binding.

Here is the list of fruits to eat and drink in the order of priority.

1. Fruits at 100% Acid Binding – Best fruits To Eat And Drink : Lemons, melons – any type, watermelon
2. Fruits at 93% Acid Binding – Great fruits To Eat And Drink
3. Cantaloupes, dried dates, dried figs, limes, mango, papaya
4. Fruits at 87% Acid Binding – Still Great Fruits To Eat And Drink Kiwis, passion fruit, pineapples, raisins, umeboshi plums
5. Fruits at 80% Acid Binding – Eat And Drink These Fruits
6. Apricots, avocados, bananas, fresh dates, fresh figs, currants, gooseberries grapes, grapefruits guavas, kumquats, nectarines, pears, persimmons, quince
7. Fruits at 73% Acid Binding – Still Fruits To Eat And Drink
   Apples, organs, peaches, pomegranate, raspberries, sour grapes, strawberries
8. Fruits at 67% Acid Binding – Still Neutralizes Acids, Eat And Drink This fruit
   Cherries

Fruits To Concentrate On

These are the fruits you should concentrate on eating. Also eat them every day, if possible, fresh lemon juice in the morning, watermelon during the day.

You can see which fruits give you the best acid binding effects and eating and drinking them 80% of your overall food intake will convert your body over to an Alkaline body.

Chapter 9: How Juices Bring Better Health

Here are some of the fruits that I listed in the previous lesson. I give you information on some of the best fruit juices to use.

Use them between meals, before meals, in some cases, or just before bedtime. You can also drink the juices that are listed in the previous lesson that are not listed here. The important thing is you can target certain juices for specific illness, or use them as a general body tonic. Use a variety of juices to get the benefit of the different nutrients that these fruit juices have.

Juices are powerful remedies and sources of quick health. They are concentrated in their nutrients and are quickly, within minutes, absorbed into your blood, since they require little or no digestion. For this reason you can use them to rebuild, cleanse, and detoxify your body quickly and easily.

Juices can help you prevent, retard, or cure illness. However, they must be used properly and at the right times. In some cases, use of juices as a therapy can have side effects, but when used in moderation they have little side effects. There are certain fruit juices that are high in natural sugars, so if you have diabetes, it is best to avoid them. If you have sensitive throats or respiratory issue, then you should not use citrus juices. And, there are also some people that are allergic to specific fruits.

All diseases respond to the use of specific fruit juices because they correct and rebalance the heat or cold in the body. They remove and neutralize toxins. So, use them when you have a fever or when you have a cold.

It is always best to juice those fruits that are grown locally. The nutrients supplied by these fruits are related to the surrounding climate and environment and provide you with the nutrients that you need. It is ok to drink exotic juices like mango, pineapple, guava, and other tropical juices, but these should be kept to around 20% of the juices you drink.

At times, juices can pull out too many toxins from your body, if you are too toxic, causing you to feel sick and uneasy. Some people get an upset stomach, if they drink juices the first thing in the morning. I suspect that this happens because juices are detoxifying the stomach and gastrointestinal tract.

Juice side effects can range from headaches to rashes or pain. Side effects will subside as you drink the juices and continue to detoxify your body.

Fresh juices are easy to create with a juicer and give you the pleasure of knowing you are giving your body the nutrients it needs. They give you a quick lift because of the nutrients and the natural sugar they contain. Once in your mouth, nutrients and sugar immediately enter your blood and are delivered soon after into your cells. This is why they are good for people who are recovering from an illness or are trying to re-develop good health.

Always use fresh juice when possible. One glass of juice can count as more than one serving of fruit. Bottled juice no longer has the pH that fresh juice has and loses a slight amount of its pH value. This means bottled juice may be acidic instead of alkaline.

However when certain juices are not available fresh, it is always best to use bottled or packaged juice to preserve your health.

Avoid buying juices in cans, aluminum containers, and plastic bottles. These juices have been highly processed and tend to have reduced nutritional value.

Chapter 10: Fruit Juices For Weight Loss

Juice Equipment

For most fruits you need to use a juice extractor. But for citrus fruits – oranges, grapefruit, lemons, and limes – it is best to use a citrus press to squeeze the juice out manually. Then you can also remove the pulp and put it into the juice, if you like. Most citrus fruits will clog up a juice extractor unless it is specifically made for citrus.

Juicer prices run from $50 to $1000. For the very best juicer, you will have to put out around $200 to $400. You will not need one of those high price juicers unless you are running a business. If you decided that juicing is going to be your life, then you need a good juicer priced around $250.

Here are the four most popular types of juicers – masticating, centrifugal, triurating, and press. Each one has advantages and you have to decide what benefits and features you want from a juicer. You can go on the internet a do a search for each one to see which one will fit your needs.

Using Juices

Once you create your juice, you should drink it right away.
If you plan to take it to work, add a teaspoon of vitamin C powder or the juice of half lemon to act as a preservative. Store the thermos in the refrigerator, if possible. If not possible, then consume the juice with a couple of hours.

The amount of juice that you should use is dependent on many items. For weight loss, you want to drink those juices that contain more fiber. Normally, juicing remove most of the fiber, except some of the more expensive juicer maintain the fiber in your juice.

Drinking juices will help you lose weight. The reason is that juices help your remove acid and waste from your body. Acid and waste is sometimes converted over to fat.

Choosing Your Fruits

Always try to get your fruits fresh and in season at a farmers market. I always ask the vendor "when was your fruit picked?" Some times you get a straight honest answer, but not all of the time. At least you let the vendor know that bringing the recent picked fruits to market gets him the most customers and sales.

Wash fruits and peel them if necessary. Remove any bruised, contaminated, or decayed areas before juicing. Core and remove seeds from most fruits.

Fruits to Use

In one of the chapters is a list of which fruits are best for turning an acid body to an alkaline body. These are the fruits that you should use and eat. Keep in mind that one juice may help one person for a particular condition and for another it may not help at all. But, in general, juices are a powerful way to recover health.

Lemons

Before juicing lemons roll then on a table top to get them slightly soft. Lemons added to other juices give them additional flavor or soften their sweetness or saltiness. Lemons are antiseptic and act as a powerful cleanser for the entire body. You can take a small sip of lemon juice before a meal to cleanse your stomach and the small intestine.

Drinking lemon juice with warm water in the morning is useful in restoring chemical balance in your body. It restores the positive and negative chemical ions in your body to a more natural state. In addition, it helps the liver create many different digestive enzymes. This results in you digesting your food better and gives you an increase in energy.

Since lemon juice, just like other citrus juices, contain a high level of minerals and potassium they are especially good to drink, without sugar, during heavy work, sports, workouts, or competitive sports.

You can mix the juices of lemon, lime, oranges, and pineapple. They all have a cleansing effect on your body. They purge and eliminate wastes from your body. You can reduce the effects of diseases such as heart, arthritis, diabetes, high blood pressure, cancer, and many other degenerative diseases by using these 4 juices together or singly. These juices will also help you lose weight.

Lime

Lime has as similar nutritional value as oranges, but less. Lime is an excellent juice to use to recover health. But, it should be used in moderate amounts. Mixed with lemon juice, it creates a powerful healing juice. It acts as a general tonic for the whole body by energizing, restoring, and rejuvenating. It flushes out toxins and wastes from your body and re-energizes your organs.

When you wake up in the morning, put 6 oz. of distilled water into a blender, slightly warm is better but room temperature is ok. Press out the juice of one lemon and one lime and put the juice and meat into the blender. Spike with a touch of cayenne pepper. Blend for 1 minute, and then drink this powerful healing juice.

Oranges

Never keep oranges in the refrigerator, since they lose their nutritional value. Squeeze your oranges in a manual orange press to get the most juice.

Oranges improve the skin complexion, assists in constipation, acts as a mild laxative, removes toxins and wastes from the body, acts as a diuretic and improves your vision.

A glass of orange juice in the morning will activate your digestion, improve your health, and give you a feeling of well being. Drinking a small amount after meals improves your digestion. It can be used in low amounts by diabetics.

Papayas

Papaya juice is a highly curative fruit and its juice gives a powerful punch for health. It keeps arteries soft and flexible, preventing the deposition of cholesterol. Its digestive enzyme, pepsin, destroys the outer layer of germs, including the TB bacteria. It reduces the risk of high blood pressure, heart attacks, and improves the circulation of blood, improves liver function, restores peristaltic intestinal action, and improves vision.

It is good for the aged, since it will improve their digestion allowing more nutrients to get into their body. It is a powerful meat digestive enzyme. You can use this in small amounts when eating meat protein.

Mango Juice

Mango is another health winner. Its juices help to build muscles and to strengthen tissue. It is an excellent heart and brain tonic. It is useful in constipation, digestive issues, reducing phlegm and acidity. It can expel worms, acts as an aphrodisiac, and blood rejuvenator and purifier.

Mix one part milk with 2 parts mango juice or puree and 4 parts water. You can use another juice instead of milk, since milk causes mucus formation.

Apples

Because apples have a high mineral content they are especially good for your skin, hair and fingernails. Apples that are good for juices are Granny Smith, Braeburn, Egremont Russet, and Discovery. You can also juice Gala apples. If they are firm and crisp they provide good juice. When buying apple juice, buy juice that is cloudy and not clear. The cloudy juice has more fiber and nutrients and contains a good amount of the fiber pectin.

Apple juice serves as a good base when mixed with other juices and especially with vegetables. Most of the vitamins lie in the skin of the apple, so it is best to juice apples without peeling.

This is one of the fruits that can be used in many ways and you still get it nutritional value. You can eat it raw, cooked, baked, juiced, jammed, or pickled.

Grape Juice

Add grape juice to other juices like apple to give it a different flavor. When juicing apples, you can juice a few handfuls of grapes also. Grapes have a high content of natural sugar and can give you a quick energy lift. They contain a high level of minerals and have B vitamins. You can drink this juice from bottles, since it has a short season and in a bottle you can drink it any time. Use the darker grape drinks, because of their high anti-oxidant nutrients

Grapes help to regulate and increase your metabolism. A low metabolism will cause you to gain weight and a high metabolism will help you burn food quicker.

Cherries

Fresh cherry juice is a powerful body alkalizer and reduces the acidity in your blood and tissues. It is an excellent remedy to reduce and eliminate gout pain. Gout is an excess of acid in the joints and tissue and results from eating too much protein. Drinking this juice between meals will help activate peristaltic bowel action, which can help to keep you regular

Melons, Cantaloupes

All melons create super juices filled with the best nutrient your body can have. They are at the top of the list for making your body more alkaline. They are good for your skin and provide your nerves with the right nutrients. Melons have a cooling effect on the body and improve your digestion.

Watermelon

Watermelon juice can be obtained by simply eat raw watermelon, since it is 98% distilled water. Its use helps cleanse the kidney and bladder, since it is a diuretic – removes excess fluids from the body. You can chew on the seeds as you eat watermelon to get the extra zinc and vitamin E

Watermelon juice tones your body, prevents heat stroke, normalizes high blood pressure, and strengthens your heart and brain. It improves digestion, calms the nerves, and is a mild laxative.

Eat watermelon in the morning. Its juice will help you remove nightly accumulated toxin through your urine. This will you restore kidney function.

Pineapple Juice

Pineapple juice is another excellent juice to use frequently. Its high potassium helps to keep your nerve transmissions active. Its health value comes from its enzyme bromelain. Bromelain helps keep your body fluids balanced and neutral; moves an acid body to neutral and an alkaline one to neutral.

When making pineapple juice do not juice the center core, since it contains some harmful chemicals. You can drink pineapple juice just before a meal as an appetizer. You can also drink it 10 – 15 minutes after a meal. It helps rejuvenate and cleanse your body. It also acts as a laxative so it helps to reduce constipation.

It is a juice and fruit to be avoided by pregnant women or women trying to get pregnant, since it contracts the uterus.

Pomegranate

Pomegranate juice controls bile and phlegm, increases hemoglobin and purifies blood, improves appetite, and settles upset stomachs. It restores and sharpens memory, and is effective in urinary issues. It is helpful in many diseases, since it neutralizes body acids.

Chapter 11: Preparing Smoothies For Weight Loss

Creating Health Smoothies

Fruit smoothies provide you a different way to eat fruits and drink their juices. Smoothies mixed with other power ingredients and nutrients can serve to give you better health and help your lose weight. Smoothies can be used to build, cleanse, and heal your body.

In cases where you are depleted of various vitamins and minerals, smoothies are a way to bring these nutrients quickly into your body. When you follow the Body Cycles, smoothies have a place as part of your morning breakfast.

Because the blender grinds down the fruits you use and mixes them with any juices you use, your body will absorb this mixture much faster then when eating the solid fruit.

The smoothies listed here also provide you with plenty of fiber. Fiber is one of the main foods you want to increase in your success eating habits program, so that you can lose weight.

Drink your smoothie slowly. Do not drink it like water. The best way to drink it is to move the mixture around in your mouth so saliva is mixed with the smoothie ingredients. Drinking a smoothie too fast can lead to gas (air in the smoothie) to form in the stomach and intestine, which can cause some discomfort.

Once your smoothie is made, drink it within a few minutes. The smoothie ingredients will start to oxidize and decay quickly as it has air mixed in from the blending process. If you fill a thermos to the top, you can use the smoothie for later, but it is always best to add a teaspoon or more of powdered vitamin C to act as a preservative.

Use fresh fruit when possible. Fresh juices will provide you with a mixture that will add more minerals to your body and thereby making your body's pH more alkaline.

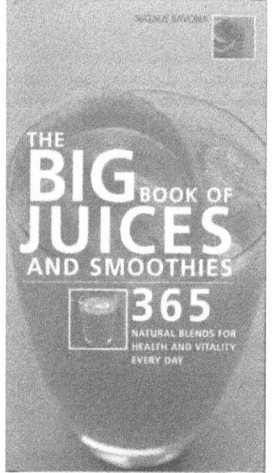

In her book, The Big Book of Juices and Smoothies, 2003, Natalie Savona, gives some hints on storing your smoothie.

"There really is no such thing as storing a juice or smoothie – you can't beat drinking them the moment you've made them. However, you may like to take them out to work or on a picnic. In that case, the best way to store them is to put a teaspoon of vitamin C powder or a squeeze of lemon juice in the bottom of the jug attached to the juicer.

The vitamin C acts as an antioxidant, preventing the juice from turning brown. The same goes for smoothies. Also keep the drinks covered and cool – in a sealed container in the refrigerator, or in a thermos flask"

Smoothie Base

Here is how you build a smoothie that can help you lose weight and give you health benefits. The smoothie base is liquid slurry that can be used to add more ingredients.

The liquid base can be made from various fresh juices or rice, oat, or almond milks. I stay away from milk since milk creates mucus along the gastrointestinal lining and contains saturated fat. Under a maintenance diet, you can add small amounts of milk to what you eat.

Choose and mix any of the following liquid and pour them into a blender.

Juices – apple, pineapple, orange, tangerine, lemon
Milks – rice dream, oat milk, almond milk

You can use a combination of 40% rice dream, 40% almond milk, and 20% apple juice. You can use any combination you like. For losing weight, for the first 10 days, use 80% apple juice and 20% of the other types of juices or milks.

Banana Base

Next, I always put in a banana. This gives the liquid a bit more thickness. Also bananas are high in potassium and other minerals. Use bananas that are not overripe since they have too much sugar. Do not use under ripe bananas, since they will create acid in your body, as well as all other fruits that are not ripe and ready to eat.

Main Ingredients

Next I choose a fruit that will be the main ingredient so you can say you are making a strawberry smoothie or a blueberry smoothie. If you have fresh organic fruit, then this is the best way to create your smoothie. You can freeze fruits during its season so I can have some of this fruit a bit long than its seasonal run. Choose from fruits that are in season.

Avocado (use sparingly)
Cantaloupe, watermelon
Peach, mango, papaya, guava
Pineapple, apricots, apples
Strawberries, blueberries, raspberries
Figs dried prunes, peaches, apricots, figs

More Nutrients to Add

Once you have your basic smoothie, you can add other

nutrients that will provide you with additional fiber, oil, vitamins, minerals and many other nutrients.

Here is a shortlist of some of the ingredients you can add to your smoothies. Add only 2-3 other ingredients so the tastes don't get to complex or unusual.

Almonds (grind to a powder with a coffee grinder)
Beet Juice powder
Capra mineral whey
Chia Seeds
ROI water Ice cubes
Edible dairy whey
Fig Juice syrup
Flaxseed and flax seed oil
Honey, rice syrup
Lecithin granules
Powder vitamin C
Raisins
Rice or oat bran
Sesame seeds
Sunflower seeds, pumpkin seeds
Wheat germ

A nice powder to add to your smoothie is called Ruby Reds. It adds a powerful punch to your smoothies, since it contains the powder of 35 fruit powders. This gives your smoothie a boost of vitamins, minerals, probiotics, antioxidants, photonutrients, and digestive enzymes. It's an excellent blend, and you can use with each smoothie.

Make sure you add a tablespoon or more of lecithin granules. This helps to keep your arteries clean and blood thinner. Lecithin also has choline which helps to create acetylcholine a neurotransmitter for your brain. Lecithin is used in every cell of your body and is a necessary nutrient.

You can also add bran and whole seeds into the blender and it will break them up, if it is a high speed blender.

Chapter 12: Health Smoothie Recipes You Will Love

So, here are a few smoothie recipes you can blend. Just use the ideas presented in the previous chapter to build up your smoothies. Drink these smoothies for breakfast or take them to work for snack time.

Apple Smoothie
Apple-Barley Smoothie
Apricot Smoothie
Peach-Rice Dream Smoothie
Pineapple Smoothie
Strawberry Smoothie
Sweet-Yams-Banana Smoothie
Papaya Smoothie
Prune and Apple Juice Blend
Banana Fig Smoothie
High Fiber Breakfast Smoothie
Mango Cool Smoothie
Mango Passion Smoothie
Papaya Smoothie

Apple Smoothie

Mix in the blender the following.

1-2 small apples cut into wedges
1 banana
1 cup 50:50 rice dream: almond milk
¼ cup or less of raisins soaked overnight
1-teaspoon honey
1-2 cubes of ice
1-teaspoon lecithin granules

2 teaspoons flax seed oil

Start by mixing the banana and the liquids. Then add slices of apples to get the consistency you like.

Apricot Smoothie

One cup of fresh apricots or dried apricots that were soaked overnight

Juice of 1/2 a lemon
Two oz. of prune juice
One teaspoon or more of oat ban
One teaspoon of mineral whey

Add a slight amount of distilled water to make the consistency to your liking.

Peach-Rice Dream Smoothie

Mix in the blender:

2 fresh peaches with peel
1-cup rice dream or almond milk
1/2 banana
1-teaspoon sesame seeds
1-teaspoon sunflower seed
1-teaspoon lecithin granules
2 teaspoons flax seed oil

Pineapple Smoothie

Mix the following in a blender.

1-2 cups of fresh pineapples
1/2 cups apple slices
1/4 cup fresh apple juice
1/2 cup apple juice (more or less as needed)
1 banana

1-teaspoon lecithin
1-teaspoon flax seeds
2 teaspoons bran (wheat, oat or rice)

Strawberry Smoothie

Mix in a blender the following ingredients.

1 banana
1-teaspoon of lecithin granules
1-teaspoon of any type of bran
1 cup or more 50:50 rice dream: almond milk
Now add strawberries one by one with the blender on until you get the consistency you like.
Now in a coffee grinder, grind the following and add them to the blended strawberry mix:
1-teaspoon flax seeds
1 or 2 teaspoon sunflower seeds
1-teaspoon sesame seeds

Prune and Apple Juice Blend

Rinse prunes in distilled water to remove any dirt or contamination. Soak 3/4 cup or more of prunes overnight. Just slightly cover the prunes with distilled water. In the morning, blend prunes with its water and one cup of apple juice. Add a couple slices of apple with its peel. Squeeze 1/2 lemon and blend again.

Add more apple juice to get the consistency you like.
This makes a great morning drink to get your bowels moving later in the morning.

Banana Fig Smoothie

Use 1 cup of rice dream, almond milk, and soymilk mixture. You can use just one of these liquids or all combined. Add one banana and figs to get the thickness you like.

After you have blended this mixture add the following:

1 teaspoon of sesame seeds
1 teaspoon or more of lecithin
1 teaspoon or more of flaxseed oil

This mixture will give you many minerals and nutrients and in addition help as a natural laxative drink

High Fiber Breakfast Smoothie

Here's a drink you can prepare in the morning and can serve as breakfast.

In a blender add,
One half a banana that is not overripe
One half an apple
A few strawberries, fresh or frozen
¾ cup or so of rice dream, almond milk, or organic soymilk
one rounded teaspoon of each bran - wheat, rice, and oat.
one tablespoon of lecithin granules
one teaspoon of flaxseed oil

The bran will help you bulk up your stool.

Mango Cool Smoothie

Combine the following in a blender:
One peeled and cored mango
1/4 to 1/2 cup of orange juice
1/2 banana
a few ice cubes to give it some consistency
teaspoon of flaxseed oil
teaspoon to tablespoon of oat bran
teaspoon of sesame seeds

Chapter 13: Step By Step Details For Losing Weight

In any diet you can lose weight. But there always seems to be a problem after the diet where 90% of dieters gain their weight back in a year.

So what is the solution for not gaining weight back? The solution is not to think you are dieting, but creating a new eating habit. But at the start of this program, the way to eat is more restrictive, so that you can start to lose weight right away. Then after ten days you can start eating food that was restricted during your first ten days.

You don't have to be so strict with all the ideas and steps that are outlined for you. But, the more you are, the more weight you will lose.

I have given you a lot of information on how you can lose weight and regain and keep healthy. All of this information can be confusing and you may have some problems trying to figure out what to do with all of this.

This e-book has provided you with some complex information that you can use to create an eating lifestyle that you can use for the rest of your life. With this new eating habit, your will be able to lose weight and then maintain your weight. If you happen to gain a little weight then just tighten up on what you eat and you will lose weight again.

Here is a program that you can use to help you get started.

An Eating Habits Lifestyle For Losing Weight And Keeping It Off

Step 1 – Colon and Blood Cleansing Diet

Doing a body cleanse at the start of this program is important and this is the first thing you need to do. A cleanse of this type should be done once a year. Here are a few things this cleanse does for you.

Cleans out your colon of any toxins
Helps to get your bowel movements back to normal
Removes some toxins from your cells and lymph liquid
Removes excess water from your body

Moves your body away from an acid body making it more alkaline

Uses some of your fat to provide you with energy during your cleanse.

Step 2 – Using Your Body Cycles

Once you finish your cleanse, you are ready to start your new eating pattern. Using the Body Cycles will help you detoxify your body daily, lose weight, keep your weight off, and improve your health.

You are ready to start practicing Body Cycle 1

This cycle is from the time you get up to noon time. During this time you only want to eat fruits and vegetables and drink juices and teas. This cycle helps you get rid of toxins that your body has accumulated during the night. It does this by urine and bowel movements. You can help your body by providing liquid and nutrients to help detoxify it.

Morning Drink

I have outlined the different drinks that you can use during this time. Here is a summary of these different types of drinks When you first get up, drink one of the following drinks. Each day you can choose a different drink or you can change every week to get the benefits of the different drinks.

a. Eight oz. of water with one lemon juice – detoxifies the liver

b. Eight oz. of water with one lemon juice and 1 to 3 tablespoons of chlorophyll liquid – improves blood and detoxifies the stomach, intestines, blood, and colon.

c. A tea of ginger – improves blood circulation

d. A cup of green tea – helps to detoxify your body and is good for your cardiovascular system.

e. A glass of a mixture of 3 citrus fruits. With a hand juicer, prepare a mixture of one orange, one grapefruit, and one lemon – helps to detoxify the body and starts eliminating acids from your body. Use this drink only once or twice a week.

f. A glass of tomato juice with the juice of one lemon – provides lycopene, anti-oxidants, and builds blood - helps you to lose weight.

g. Take a glass of green drink. You can buy some super green powders that contain all kinds of nutrients and plenty of green vegetable power. Add some honey to sweeten the taste. Some of these green drinks don't taste so good.

Shower Time

After your morning drink go take a shower and get dressed. After you do this you are ready for the next step.

Morning Fruit

Now you are ready to have some fruit, fruit pudding, vegetable juice, or morning shake. Vary what you eat at this point so that you can give your body a variety of nutrient that will help to promote a good bowel movement. You can chose from the following list of what you want to eat.

a. Slices of watermelon, cantaloupes, or any other type of melon. You can mix them together – helps to eliminate acids from your body and promotes urine.

b. A bowl of different fruit such as apple, mango, pineapple, strawberries, and berries. Chose those fruits on the list provided that will provide you with a lot of fiber – fiber will help you lose weight and keeps your colon clean. Remember you need to eat up to 30 to 35 grams of fiber in this eating habits program.

c. A bowl of the special soup as outlined in the previous chapter. This soup you can eat anytime that you get hungry. So, you will want to take some to work in a thermos. The liquid and vegetables will help to promote a bowel movement.

d. A pudding of different fruits that you put in a blender. Add some apple juice or other juices you like to adjust the pudding consistency – helps to give you fiber, make your body more alkaline, and activates peristaltic action for a bowel movement.

e. A smoothie as outline in the previous chapter. Use this type of smoothie only 1 or 2 times a week – fiber and special nutrients help you to lose weight and to keep you healthy.

You can use your own ideas of how you want to eat fruits and vegetables at this time. I have just given you some ideas to start.

Step 3 - Morning Snack

Usually morning snack time is around 10 am. At this time you want to have the following type of snacks.

a. Eat the special soup that you have prepared and that is in your thermos.

b. Eat more fruit like apples, strawberries, or watermelon – helps reduce body acid, provides fiber, and helps you to eliminate body toxins through urine and stools.

c. Drink some leftover smoothie that you brought in a thermos.

d. Drink some juice that was mentioned in the previous chapter – helps to promote bowel movements and keep your body alkaline.

There you have it. You can see that your morning should be devoted to helping your body get rid of toxins by not blocking your digestion process with heavy food. Eggs, bread, meat, and other heavy carbohydrates take around 3 to 4 hours to digest. When you eat these foods your detoxification process stops or is slowed down. This keeps you fat.

Eating fruits and vegetables take around 1 to 2 hours to digest. This helps to pushes toxins out of your body in the morning. This is the time when your body is working to get rid of night toxins and poisons. Help your body do its work and you will lose weight.

Step 4 - Lunch Time

Noon is the time to eat heavy food. It is this food that is going to give you the nutrients to provide your body with energy and to help it regenerate itself.

For lunch you want to only eat enough food for your daily needs. When you eat more than what your body needs to keep it going, it will turn the excess into fat.

Here is some food that you should be eating for lunch.

a. Always eat a raw salad or raw vegetables with your main meal. Look at the list of vegetables and try to eat those that have the most fiber. But mix them by eating some with a lot of fiber and some with low fiber. If you eat cooked vegetables, cook them for a few minutes to minimize the degradation of the fiber.

b. You can eat all the vegetables you want from the list that is called non starchy vegetables. These vegetables will not make you gain weight.

c. Your main course can be any of the meat, poultry, or fish listed in the previous chapter. The severing size listed is not the amount you should eat. You can eat an amount to where you feel satisfied, but do not overeat. Protein can also be stored as fat, when your body does not need it. If you eat plenty during cycle 1, you will not need to eat a lot of meat at noon time. Alternate the meats you eat day after day. But always eat one type of meat for a meal.

d. The best protein to eat is fish. Beef has been found to contribute to cardiovascular diseases. So try to minimize the use of beef, if you eat it. Or, you can just reduce the serving size of beef.

e. Try to eat only one meat and vegetables – helps to improve your digestion and reduces any stomach problems. Most people are used to eating meat potatoes or rice with vegetables. If you need rice, use a reduced amount of rice.

f. Don't drink any juice or water with your lunch – improves your digestion. You can drink some room temperature water to clear your throat. Drinking a cold liquid will slow down your digestion.

g. During lunch is a good time to add a dressing to your salad. This dressing should contain some fatty oils, such as olive oil, flax oil, a small of mayonnaise. You can eat some saturated fat, since the body needs it, but do it in small amounts. Don't pour it on thick.

h. Don't eat any deserts after your lunch and especially fruits – this interrupts your digestion process. Wait about an hour before eat a desert.

Step 5 - After Lunch Snack

Use the ideas given for Morning Snacks for your after lunch snack.

Notice that you can eat many foods that you cannot in other diets. When you eat foods that you like, do it in small quantities. It is not the type of foods, with exception of processed foods since they do not fiber or enzymes, but the excess quantity of foods that you eat that make you fat.

Learn to eat less of the foods you like and eat more frequently. Always eat something during morning and afternoon snack time.

a. You can use nuts or seeds as snacks but do it in moderation – gives you some of the omega 3 and 6 fatty acids.

b. Eat some of the special soup you still have in your thermos – helps you lose weight.

c. Drink some juice like cherry juice, prune juice, apple juice or pineapple juice.

d. Eat some fruit from the list provided.

Step 6 – Dinner time

This is the time to eat carbohydrates or more protein. It is best to eat carbohydrates with vegetables and no protein. You may find this hard to do but here is what to eat at dinner time.

a. Brown rice with cooked vegetable and or a salad. You can eat all the brown rice you want, but don't over eat. If you are not use to eating without some meat add a small amount of meat to the rice.

b. You can interchange your dinner type meal with your lunch meal. Concentrate your lunch meal with carbohydrates and a little meat and at dinner concentrate on protein with a little carbohydrate.

c. Eat less meat for dinner and no fish for dinner, since meat takes a long to digest. Also, fish takes longer to digest than meat.

d. You can eat some pasta, provided you eat plenty of raw vegetables. But watch the pasta, since over eating can cause you some weight gain.

Step 7 – After Dinner Snacks

Try not to eat anything 2 to 3 hours before bedtime. If you need a snack, here is a starter list.

a. Fruits like pineapple, apple, and so on – helps to provide the minerals needed to neutralize body acids.

b. Here again you can have some vegetable soup – this soup helps you from getting or staying hungry and will not cause you to gain weight.

Final Comments

There you have it a method of changing your eating habits. So why change your eating habits? Because the way you have been eating has made you gain weight. This eating habits program is not a diet that you come off after you have lost weight, it's an eating habit that you continue to use, but in a relaxed manner, so they you can maintain your weight gain new health.

Eating differently will provide you with a different outcome – losing weight.

You don't have to stop eating a lot of the things you like you just have to eat less of them. And you need to eat healthier food. Eating an excess of processed food is a sure way to gaining and keeping weight. This type of food has no fiber and no digestive enzymes.

Follow the cycles and the foods combining that is outlined here and you will lose weight. There are a lot of foods that are listed here that you can eat, but there are some foods that you have watch and eat less of.

Chapter 14: Easy Exercises You Need for Losing Weight

You will not lose weight if you just exercise. What is most important is what you eat. Exercising is fine tuning your weight loss program. When you exercise and eat a good healthy diet you will lose weight.

Walking

So what are the exercises you should be doing? There is no need to go to the gym and spend an hour running on the tread mill or riding a bike. You can get the same benefits for your weight loss program by walking briskly any time of the day. Just set aside some walking time every day.

Other Exercises

There are many other exercises that are good for you. If you play sports and like riding a bike or swimming, then this is what you should do. Doing yoga is also an excellent exercise or dancing. You pick the exercise you like to do so that you will always look forward to do it.

The idea in losing weight is to only eat the amount of calories that your body needs or to eat just a little less than what your body needs. And, if you couple this with some exercise this will burn some more of the fat you have stored all over your body.

If you walk, walk for a comfortable distance and then either try to increase you walk every day. Or, you can walk the same distance, but walk it faster.

Rebounder

Using a rebounder is another way to exercise at home. With the rebounder you can jump up and down and help tone your muscles. In addition, you activate the lymph liquid in your body to circulate better. This is an excellent way to help your body detoxify, especially if you do this in the morning.

Actually, doing your exercise in the morning will definitely help your body detoxify and help you lose more weight.

The Pace Program

There is another program that is one of the best exercise programs that is available. It is called the "PACE" exercise program. You can learn more about this on the internet. This program is great for losing weight and for strengthening your cardiovascular system.

Chapter 15: About The Author And Other Resources

Rudy Silva is a natural consultant nutritionist educated in the United State in Nutrition and Physics. He is a graduate from the San Jose State University in California. He is author of 30 other e-books on natural remedies. He has authored a newsletter in natural remedies for over 4 years. He has many websites promoting special recommended products and information.

Resource page

Here are some of the other kindle e-books about natural remedies that have been written by this author.

Acne Remedies

Natural Help With Acne
Best natural acne treatments: Acne facial

Constipation Remedies

The Best Constipation Remedies
Best Constipated Women Natural Cures
How To Relieve Constipation With Fruits

Essential Fatty Acids

Taking The Mystery Out Of Essential Fatty acids
Amazing Fish Oil Benefits Revealed

Nutrition Remedies

Updated Version - Secret Diet And Nutrition

Secret Healthy Fruit Practices Revealed
Fast Healing Juice Nutrition Therapy: Nutrition Tips 3
Fantastic Alkaline Fruit Benefits Revealed
Calcium (Discover How To Use Calcium To Avoid Devastating Diseases)
Magnesium Nutrition Revealed
Best Nutrition Health Practices
Potassium Health Secrets Revealed
Phosphorus, The Best Brain Food

Stomach Remedies

Acid Reflux: Fast and Easy Cures For Acid Reflux
Asthma Treatment Cures With Remedies
How To Do Natural Colon Cleansing
Gastrointestinal Digestion Secrets Revealed

Misc Remedies

Natural Hair Loss Treatment: Women And Men
Effective Natural Hemorrhoids Treatment
Iron Deficiency Anemia
Secrets To Understanding Behavior
Fast Acting Ear Infection Remedies
Best Impotence Health Diet
What Is A Hiatus Hernia
Best Varicose Vein Treatments?

To see all of the kindle books written by this author, go to this the **Authors Profile Page**.

If you need support or want to promote any of his e-books, please contact him at **rss41@yahoo.com** and expect a reply within 24 hours. He looks forward to hearing from you and is happy to help you understand his material on natural and nutritional health.

Give A Review

And, don't for get to give a review for this e-book at Amazon so that others can gain the benefits of what is in this e-book.

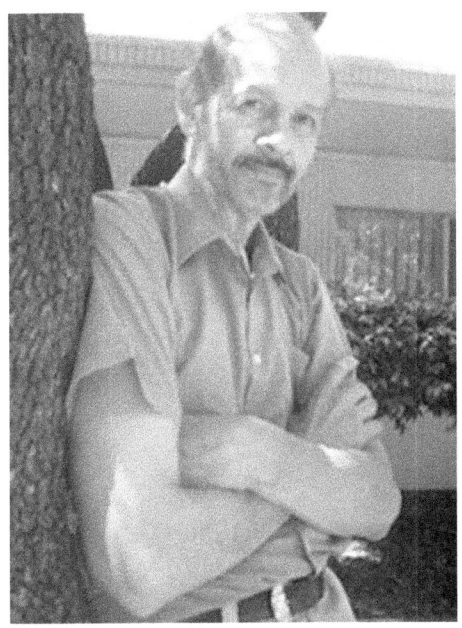

To you, for losing weight, creating better health and more happiness in your life,

Rudy S Silva

www.ingramcontent.com/pod-product-compliance
Lightning Source LLC
Chambersburg PA
CBHW070559290526
45790CB00002B/735